Reversing Polycythemia Vera Naturally

The Raw Vegan Plant-Based Detoxification & Regeneration Workbook for Healing Patients.

Volume 2

I0090531

Health Central

Copyright © 2023

Topics Discussed & Journal Structure

1. Naturally Healing Your Polycythemia Vera

2. Our Story

3. Important Notes for Overcoming Your Polycythemia Vera

4. The Power of Journaling

5. Daily Journal Examples

6. Frequently Asked Questions (Vol.2)

7. 30 Day Assisted Journal Section

Naturally Healing Your Polycythemia Vera

"Let food be thy medicine and medicine be thy food."

- Hippocrates

Throughout this series of journals, we discuss a tried and tested healing protocol that we discovered through the healing of our own ailments and conditions.

The aim is to increase your internal Oxygen levels, alkalize your body, cleanse your digestive and lymphatic systems (and blood) whilst increasing your absorption and energy levels. Good health will soon follow, and this is our ultimate goal because "diseases" cannot exist within healthy individuals.

As we know, all species originally ate raw. Fruits and some vegetables were the foods intended for our (Fruigivore) species. Our evolution into food mixing and constantly eating the wrong/"junk" cooked foods has lead to today's "disease" crisis. Cooked/low energy foods (mainly animal and starch based) hinder healing and create the perfect environment for sickness to exist.

An internal alkaline environment on the other hand (achieved mainly through fruits and vegetables) repels disease, suffering and pain, whilst encouraging healing and regeneration.

Having healed ourselves and helped many others – we have arrived at a series of conclusions and treatment protocols:

1.   Regardless of the labelled "condition" or "disease" – the obstruction of an internal acidic environment can be

corrected. For example, if your car has an oil leak, you don't just stick a plaster over the leak. Instead you find the root cause and repair this. Similarly we want to correct our root issues in order to achieve lasting results.

2. In simple terms, "dis-ease" within the body stems from internal congestion resulting from the sustained consumption of acid-forming (cooked) foods which the body struggles to process.

3. Our lymphatic system is responsible for washing our blood but when it has become stagnant/un-responsive, the acids just continue to slowly pile up in our blood. With our organs now surrounded by "un-washed" blood, dis-ease begins.

4. For us to activate our lymphatic system, we need to initiate filtration of our skin and kidneys (your skin being the 3rd kidney and largest eliminative organ – through sweat). Regular bowel movements also support the detoxification process. The combination of herbs, intermittent dry fasting and eating/juicing fruit will regulate these systems.

5. Sleep is important and allows for recovery. We advise patients to sleep from 10pm every night and awaken when it feels natural to do so. Be sure to stop all eating by early evening so your body can start to wind down and prepare for sleep.

6. Dry fasting (nil by mouth) eliminates toxins and weak cells that are not performing at their best. Intermittent fasting has helped many patients achieve positive results. Dry fast until as late as possible into the day before eating a fruit that additionally has a laxative effect (e.g. prunes,

plums, grapes, figs, oranges). This process will help flush out the fast's accumulated toxins. Hyrdration is very important here.

IMPORTANT NOTE: after a long dry fast, a "laxative fruit" (prunes, grapes, mangos) is necessary because fasts can cause constipation. Another key point with dry fasting is that you MUST hydrate well upon breaking your fast. Drink plenty of water (spring water where possible), eat plenty of water-dense fruit such as mangos, apples, citrus fruits (grapefruit, orange, clementine), berries, or melons.

7. Long dry fasts do yield great results but they can be harsh on your adrenal glands (stressful) and kidneys so we advise taking kidney and adrenal glandulars and/or herbs such as liquorice root, manjistha, stinging nettle to support them both. The longer you can dry fast, whilst limiting your eating window, the better the results will be. However, you must work up to this. **DO NOT** just jump in with a long dry fast. Start by having a delayed fruit breakfast, working towards skipping breakfast altogether, to having only 1 fruit meal in the day (with some vegetables every so often for re-mineralisation). Always work at your own pace and listen to your body. Again, drinking plenty of water after fasting is important. Be sure to remain balanced with dry fasting as it can lead to dehydration and potential binge eating if left unmonitored.

Critical Notes: Fruit coupled with fasting will expose your weaknesses so you will need to be prepared for this. Your body will eliminate all past illnesses that may have been suppressed with allopathic medicines, along with other toxic loads. This can be quite an experience so having the appropriate supplementation in place to support your detox is crucial. Consuming herbs (dandelion root, milk thistle, cleavers, astragalus, stinging nettle, parsley) is recommended for all pre-existing weaknesses. Vegetables will support a slower detoxification whilst feeding your cells healing nutrients.

Iridology Session: We would recommend having your main weaknesses identified through an Iris Diagnosis session. This will help you to focus and prioritise your goals. Search for reliable and well known Iridologists (Dr Robert Morse's clinic offers this service) that work off the Dr Bernard Jensen model. We found these sessions to be a supportive and revealing part of healing.

8. The goal is to work up towards completing 7 consecutive days of fruit fasting (it becomes significantly easier from this point on) and then to 14 days, 30 days, and so on. The balance between fruits and vegetables/salads is something that you will need to experiment with and find what works best for you. For us, we found that eating fruit for breakfast and lunch, and vegetables/salads for dinner worked well for us.

9. As parasites and various other toxic elements die off, you may experience certain symptoms. One common symptom is extreme food cravings (for starchy/meaty/cheesy foods) – but do not be fooled, this is not YOU craving, it is just the parasites trying to pull you back down and resisting your cleansing attempts. You could take some parasite cleansing herbs (wormwood, clove, black wallnut) to aide their removal.

10. Fruit (e.g. melons, berries, grapes, citrus) with the rich fructose content will be your main food during your detoxification period. For the deepest detox experience, slow juice your fruits and stick with a single fruit throughout (grape juice alone has given us the best results – oranges are also very impressive).

11. Juicing allows for accelerated results (your body can focus all of its energy on healing as opposed to digestion). Specific herbs (e.g. Cleavers, Manjistha, Parsley, Cilantro) will enhance detoxification. Vegetables are very good for providing minerals and nutrients to your healing body and they slow down the rate of detoxification which could be a requirement if you are experiencing severe detoxification symptoms. Keep in mind that starches, nuts/seeds, legumes, and cooked foods will halt the detoxification process.

Note: Proteins, dairy, and grain-based foods will reverse your detoxification progress so these foods need to be eliminated from your diet.

12. Dried fruits (dates, figs, apricots, bananas, avocados) can be used to assist if you are feeling empty or struggling with cravings in the initial stages. However, do get back onto water-dense fresh/tree-ripened fruit (watermelons/melons, berries, oranges, and grapes being the preferred kind) as soon as possible (ideally juiced). A list of detox-proven fruits can be found in the following point.

13. Examples of fruits proven to offer reliable hydration and detoxification include: Apples, Apricots, Blueberries, Blackberries, Cherries, Clementines, Figs, Tangerines, Lemons, Limes, Grapefruit, Mango, Grapes, Strawberries,

Raspberries, Oranges, Pomegranates, Pineapples, Plums, Pears, Prunes, Watermelon

14. It is important that your body is absorbing correctly otherwise deficiencies can ensue. We have found most patients to be suffering from malabsorption – this is confirmed through the iris. In this case, we must focus on cleansing the intestinal walls. In the meantime, it is advised to correct any deficiencies through supplementation where necessary.

15. If you are on medications, work with your Medical Doctor (MD) and have regular blood work done so your personal progress can be monitored. Positive results will occur within a short timeframe so do pay close attention to your state and remember to reduce medication if no longer required. We also recommend tracking your progress through an Iridology session every 6 to 12 months. This will show you which areas are resolving and those that need continued work.

Our goal throughout this workbook is to help you with recording your progress and applying the information stated in the above points. We also found that as one records progress and self journals thoughts, consciousness grows and this further encourages the achievement of goals.

Start with what you are most comfortable with and make it enjoyable, choose your favourite sweet fruits. If we ever deviated from the routine, we would help each other get back on track as soon as possible. I feel that the key is to keep moving forward, keep track of progress, and be persistent. We would like to wish you all the best. Good luck with your healing journey – it's easy - you can do it!

Our Story

It was a Sunday night, over 7 years ago – I was in bed – tossing and turning – unable to sleep. I watched the time pass, from 11pm, to 12am... to 1:30am. I just couldn't sleep. I could feel an immense pressure in my chest cavity and all across my diaphragm area. I couldn't understand where this was coming from. I got up and had some water, I then tried to use the bathroom – the discomfort was still there. Nothing seemed to work – I felt like I was being suffocated each time I would lie down. In the end, I fell asleep out of sheer fatigue.

At the time, I was a sufferer of asthma, eczema, anxiety attacks, and a damaged/leaky gut. These conditions had lead to many symptoms that doctors could not offer me any answers for. I had many tests done but nothing could tell me what the root causes of my problems were.

I started researching about my symptoms, and as I did this, I found myself expanding into the area of medical history. As my research continued, I came to understand that our ancestors lived healthy and long lives, without the health challenges of today.

Eventually, I stumbled upon a few health forums which I joined. Through these, I met a series of individuals that were battling a variety of conditions themselves (a rare genetic disorder, Crohn's disease, multiple sclerosis, muscular dystrophy (MD), diabetes, cushing's disease, a series of 'incurable' autoimmune diseases, and cancer).

We all came together and as we started to grow as a group, we made a significant discovery - that actually the cure to all diseases was discovered back in the 1920s by a Dr Arnold Ehret.

As we studied his material, we started applying his information and protocols on ourselves. This seemed like one experiment worth trying, and within 2 weeks, regardless of our individual conditions, we all started to notice a difference in our improved digestion, higher energy levels, increased mental clarity and improved physical ability. A major change was taking place – our health was improving, as our conditions were decreasing.

We continued to expand our knowledge and we started to encounter even more communities and learnt that there were more magnificent and very gifted healers out there. We came across the works and achievements of Dr Sebi, and completed an insightful and very informative course by Dr Robert Morse.

The essential message of these great healers was very similar to that of Dr Arnold Ehret. Now we had even further confirmation that the information we had been following thus far was in fact THE path to health success. With our progress so far, we could sense victory.

Within 3 months, 30 to 40 percent of our symptoms had disappeared and our health was becoming stronger. Some of us started to take specific herbs in order to enhance the detoxification.

Another 3 months on and the majority of us no longer experienced any more symptoms. Our blood work had also improved significantly, but we still had work to do in order to completely heal.

Now that we had made significant progress in reversing our conditions through self-experimentation, we started to offer basic healthy eating advice to the sick within our local communities.

Eventually, we started working with local patients on a voluntary basis. It was heartbreaking to witness lives being cut short or chronic sickness being accepted as a way of life – all whilst the lifelong eating habits of these individuals remained. The most common diseases that we were coming across included: cancers, heart disease, chronic kidney disease, high blood pressure, varying infections, and diabetes.

By helping our communities with changing their daily eating habits, we started seeing results, and although the transitional phase of moving from the foods that they were so used to eating, to moving over to a raw plant-based routine was a challenge, in the end, it was worth the shift. Note: there were many that ignored our advice and sadly they continued to remain in their state.

We did have resistance initially from family members and friends of the sick but after some time as they started seeing health improvements, more started joining us, and they also started experiencing what we had when we first set out on our journey of natural self-healing.

Nevertheless, challenges still remained – the main ones being the undoing of society's programming that cooked food is an essential part of life (including animal and wheat based products) and raw food alone surely cannot be good for you. It doesn't take long to explain how to remove imbalances and dis-ease from within the human body but the more extensive task is to actually have the protocol information applied and adhered to completely.

This is where the idea for this series of journal & progress tracker stemmed from. We felt compelled to spread this information in a more digestible and applicable form, over a series of volumes, in which we would start by offering some key informative points, followed by a journal which would allow for you to actually apply the information, record your progress, daily feelings and stay accountable to yourself. We also found that journaling and writing to oneself really helps to self-motivate and enhances a self consciousness that is needed when following a protocol like this.

Each journal volume within this series will be designed to help you record your journey for a 30 day period. At the start of each journal we will continue to offer insightful information about our experiences, whilst expanding on and re-iterating specific parts of this protocol.

The fact that you are reading this foreword is an indication that you are already on your way to self-healing. Regardless of your condition, we invite you to seek more knowledge and set your health free.

May you always remain blessed and guided.

Much Love From The Health Central Team

Important Notes for Overcoming Your Polycythemia Vera

1. It should be noted that based on our experiences and understanding, whether your condition is Polycythemia Vera, or any other, we recommend the same raw vegan healing protocol across all spectrums. With some conditions, you may need to perform a deeper detoxification (using herbs - or organ/glandular meat/capsules for more chronic situations) before achieving significant results, but in general, we have found this protocol to work in most cases. In our experience, the goal is not to cure, but instead to raise health levels first, through healthy food choices, as intended for our species – before the eradication and prevention of these modern-day "disease" conditions can take place.

2. With all conditions, we have found that the lymphatic system has become congested and overwhelmed due to the kidneys not efficiently filtering out the accumulated cell waste – as a result of years of dehydrating cooked/wheat/dairy foods. The adrenal glands work closely with the kidneys, and so adrenal/kidney herbs and glandular formulas played a major role in opening up these channels. We also found that opening up the bowels and loosening the gut was hugely important too.

3. The healing protocol that we used on ourselves is discussed and expanded upon throughout the various volumes in this series. Our goal is to share information that we have gathered from our journeys, and let you decide if it is something that you feel could also work for you in your

journey for health and vitality. You are not obliged to use this information, and you may proceed as you see fit.

Through our study, research and application, we have found this system to correct any internal imbalances and remove dis-ease that has occurred within the human body, due to the continued consumption of acid-forming foods.

4. Always take progression ultra slow and go at your own pace. Listen to your body at every stage. We cannot re-iterate this point enough. Pay attention to how you feel and continue to consult your doctor and monitor your blood work.

5. A special emphasis needs to be given to the transition phase when moving from your regular, standard diet, to a raw vegan diet that is high in fruit. You must take your time and slowly remove foods from your current routine, and replace them with either fasting or a small amount of fruit in the initial stages. Work with small amounts – please do not make any drastic changes. If you do not feel comfortable or have any concerns at any stage, please immediately stop.

Note: with any dietary change, this can be a stressful event for the body and so it is important that you support your kidneys and adrenal glands using the appropriate herbs and glandular formulas previously mentioned.

6. Before partaking in any new dietary routine, please always consult your Doctor first and ensure that they are aware of your health related goals. This approach is beneficial because (a) you can monitor your blood work with your doctor as you progress with this new protocol, and (b) if you are on any medication, as your health improves, you

can review its need and/or discuss having dosage amounts reduced (if necessary).

7. Please note that we are sharing information from our collective experiences of how we healed ourselves from a variety of diseases and conditions. These are solely our own opinions. Having reversed a range of conditions using essentially the same protocol, our understanding and conclusion, based on our experience alone, is that regardless of the disease, illness or condition name – removing it from the human body stems from correcting your diet and transitioning over to a more raw vegan lifestyle.

8. Proceed with care, and again, do not make any sudden changes – always take your time in slowly removing foods that are not serving you, and replacing them with high energy sweet tree-ripened juicy fruit. If at any point you feel that you are moving too quickly, please adjust your transition accordingly. Results may vary between individuals.

9. We recommended that you constantly expand your knowledge and familiarise yourself with the works of Dr Arnold Ehret, Dr Robert Morse and John Rose. When you feel confident with your understanding, start taking gradual steps towards reaching your goals. Make the most of this journal and use it to serve you as a companion on your journey.

The Power of Journaling

a) Journaling your inner self talk is a truly effective way of increasing self awareness and consciousness. To be able to transfer your thoughts and feelings onto a piece of paper is a truly effective method of self reflection and improvement. This is much needed when you are switching to a high fruit dietary routine.

b) Be sure to always add the date of journaling at the top of each page used. This is invaluable for when you wish to go back and review/track progress and your feelings/thoughts on previous dates.

c) Keep a comprehensive record of activities, thoughts, and really log everything you ate/are eating. You can even make miscellaneous notes if you feel that they will help you.

d) We have added tips and questions to offer you guidance, reminders, inspiration and areas to journal about.

e) We like to use journals to have a conversation with ourselves. Inner talk can really help you overcome any challenges that you are experiencing. Express yourself and any concerns that you may have.

f) Try to advise yourself as though you are your best friend – similarly to how you would advise a close friend or family member. You will be surprised at the results that you will achieve from using this technique.

g) Add notes to this journal and work your way through the 30 days. Once completed, move onto the next journal volume in this series, which will also be structured in a similar, supportive and educational fashion. We have produced a series of these journals in order to cater for your ongoing journey and goals.

h) For those of you who would like to track your progress with a more basic notebook-style journal, we have produced a separate series in which each notebook interior differs. This is to cater for your complete health journaling needs.

We have laid out the following examples to serve as potential frameworks for one way of how a journal could be filled in on a daily basis. These are just basic examples, but you can complete your daily journals in any other way that you feel is most comfortable and effective for you.

[EXAMPLE 1]
Today's Date: 2nd Jan 2020

Morning

I just ate 3 mangoes – very sweet and tasty. I felt a heavy feeling under my chest area so I stopped eating. Unsure what that was - maybe digestive or the transverse colon?

Afternoon

I was feeling hungry so I am eating some dried figs, pineapple and apricots with around 750ml of spring water.

Evening

Sipping on a green tea (herbal). Feeling pretty strong and alert at the moment.

Night

Enjoying a bowl of red seeded grapes. Currently I feel satisfied.

Today's Notes (Highlights, Thoughts, Feelings):

Unlike yesterday, today was a good day. I am noticing an increase in regular bowel movements which makes me feel cleansed and light afterwards. I feel as though my kidneys are also starting to filter better (white sediment visible in morning wee).

It definitely helps to document my thoughts in this workbook. A great way to reflect, improve and stay on track.

Feeling very good - vibrant and strong – I have noticed a major improvement in my physical fitness and performance. Mentally I feel healthier and happier.

[EXAMPLE 2]
Today's Date: 3rd Jan 2020

Morning

Dry fasting (water and food free since 8pm last night) - will go up until 12:30pm today, and start with 500ml of spring water before eating half a watermelon.

Afternoon

Kept busy and was in and out quite a bit - so nothing consumed.

Evening

At around 5pm, I had a peppermint tea with a selection of mixed dried fruit (small bowl of apricot, dates, mango, pineapple, and prunes).

Night

Sipped on spring water through the evening as required.
Finished off the other half of the watermelon from the morning.

Today's Notes (Highlights, Thoughts, Feelings):

As with most days, today started well with me dry fasting (continuing my fast from my sleep/skipping breakfast) up until around 12:30pm and then eating half a watermelon. The laxative effect of the watermelon helped me poop and release any loosened toxins from the fasting period.
I tend to struggle on some days from 3pm onwards. Up until that point I am okay but if the cravings strike then it can be challenging. I remind myself that those burgers and chips do not have any live healing energy.
I feel good in general. I feel fantastic doing a fruit/juice fast but slightly empty by the end of the day.
Cooked food makes me feel severe fatigue and mental fog.
Will continue with my fruit fasting and start to introduce fruit juices due to their deeper detox benefits. I would love to be on juices only as I have seen others within the community achieve amazing results.

[EXAMPLE 3]
Today's Date: 4th Jan 2020

Morning

Today I woke and my children were enjoying some watermelon for breakfast - and the smell was luring so I joined them. Large bowl of watermelon eaten at around 8am. Started with a glass of water.

Afternoon

Snacked on left over watermelon throughout the morning and afternoon. Had 5 dates an hour or so after.

Evening

Had around 3 mangoes at around 6pm. Felt content - but then I was invited round to a family gathering where a selection of pizzas, burgers and chips were being served. I gave into the peer pressure and felt like I let myself down!

Night

Having over-eaten earlier on in the evening, I was still feeling bloated with a headache (possibly digestion related) and I also felt quite mucus filled (wheez in chest and coughing up phlegm). Very sleepy and low energy. The perils of cooked foods!!

Today's Notes (Highlights, Thoughts, Feelings):

I let myself down today. It all started well until I ate a fully blown meal (and over-ate). I didn't remain focussed and I spun off track. As a result my energy levels were much lower and I felt a bout of extreme fatigue 30 minutes after the meal (most likely the body struggling to with digesting all that cooked food).
I need to stick to the plan because the difference between fruit fasting, and eating cooked foods is huge - 1 makes you feel empowered whilst the other makes you feel drained. I also felt the mucus overload after the meal - it kicked in pretty quickly.
Today I felt disappointed after giving in to the meal but tomorrow is a new day and I will keep on going! It is important to remind myself that I won't get better if I cannot stick to the routine.

Frequently Asked Questions (Vol.2)

Are avocados okay to eat on this protocol?

They are perfectly fine during the transition period (when moving over from cooked foods to a fruit diet). Bananas, dates and figs are another recommendation of ours. You can also make a number of tasty salads or pastas (with Zucchini/Courgette) during this period. However do keep in mind that they do not hold much detoxification value, so they should be used sparingly.

How long is the healing period - when will I be healed?

This depends on how well your body responds, how congested you were to start with – in short, a number of factors will contribute to how quickly you are able to heal. Everybody is different, some patients have had success within 30 days, whilst others have seen positive results within 60 days. Note: this is a long-term journey and we don't advise looking at timeframes but instead to focus on the positive changes that you experience - it is meant to be a lifestyle change. The rest will be down to you to decide – i.e. either continue with the routine that allows for you to feel this wonderful, or go back to low-energy foods that create fatigue and dis-ease within the body.

Can I go back to eating cooked foods?

Once you have healed and have a regular fruit routine going - if you still have a desire for a specific cooked meal, then I would say an occasional "Treat Day" wouldn't be the end of the world. However with time, you will notice a change in the foods that you desire so listen to your body. **Note:** certain cravings can stem from parasites so we tend to recommend supplementing with herbs that can support you in parasite removal (wormwood, black wallnut, clove).

Some say juicing is not good for the body – is this true?

Everybody will have different opinions so we focus on what has proven to work and achieve results. We have found juicing to be highly beneficial and patients have experienced accelerated results. Juice will deliver all of the nutrients to your body, limiting fermentation, and digestion energy. This energy will be directed towards your healing. Ensure you are drinking a sufficient amount of juice in order to receive the best level of nutrition for yourself. Everybody is unique and will have different requirements. So if you feel like you want more juice - keep juicing, but most importantly, listen to your body at all times.

30 Day Assisted Journal Section

1. Today's Date:

Morning

(work towards continuing your night time dry fast up until at least 12pm)

Afternoon

(get hydrating with fresh fruit or even better slow juiced fruits/berries/melons)

Evening

(aim to wind down to a dry fast by around 6pm to 7pm)

Night

(work your way up to dry fasting from the evening until 12pm the following day)

Today's Notes (Highlights, Thoughts, Feelings, What Could You Improve On?)

"Get yourself an accountability partner to complete a 3 month detox with.
Start with 7 days and work your way up.
It will be fun and motivating completing it with somebody (or a group) ...or of course you can go it alone"

2. Today's Date:

Morning
(work towards continuing your night time dry fast up until at least 12pm)

Afternoon
(get hydrating with fresh fruit or even better slow juiced fruits/berries/melons)

Evening
(aim to wind down to a dry fast by around 6pm to 7pm)

Night
(work your way up to dry fasting from the evening until 12pm the following day)

Today's Notes (Highlights, Thoughts, Feelings, What Could You Improve On?)

"Remember to keep yourself hydrated with water too (spring water preferred)."

3. Today's Date:

Morning
(work towards continuing your night time dry fast up until at least 12pm)

Afternoon
(get hydrating with fresh fruit or even better slow juiced fruits/berries/melons)

Evening
(aim to wind down to a dry fast by around 6pm to 7pm)

Night
(work your way up to dry fasting from the evening until 12pm the following day)

Today's Notes (Highlights, Thoughts, Feelings, What Could You Improve On?)

"Eat melons/watermelons separately, and before any other fruit as it digests faster and we want to limit fermentation (acidity) which can occur if other fruits are mixed in."

4. Today's Date:

Morning
(work towards continuing your night time dry fast up until at least 12pm)

Afternoon
(get hydrating with fresh fruit or even better slow juiced fruits/berries/melons)

Evening
(aim to wind down to a dry fast by around 6pm to 7pm)

Night
(work your way up to dry fasting from the evening until 12pm the following day)

Today's Notes (Highlights, Thoughts, Feelings, What Could You Improve On?)

"Stay focussed on the end goal of removing mucus & toxins from your body and feeling wonderful again!"

5. Today's Date:

Morning
(work towards continuing your night time dry fast up until at least 12pm)

Afternoon
(get hydrating with fresh fruit or even better slow juiced fruits/berries/melons)

Evening
(aim to wind down to a dry fast by around 6pm to 7pm)

Night
(work your way up to dry fasting from the evening until 12pm the following day)

Today's Notes (Highlights, Thoughts, Feelings, What Could You Improve On?)

"Meditate and perform deep breathing exercises in order to help yourself remain present minded and stay on track."

6. Today's Date:

Morning
(work towards continuing your night time dry fast up until at least 12pm)

Afternoon
(get hydrating with fresh fruit or even better slow juiced fruits/berries/melons)

Evening
(aim to wind down to a dry fast by around 6pm to 7pm)

Night
(work your way up to dry fasting from the evening until 12pm the following day)

Today's Notes (Highlights, Thoughts, Feelings, What Could You Improve On?)

"Join a few like-minded communities – there are many juicing and raw vegan based groups, both online and offline. Being part of a community can help motivate you to reach your goals."

---

7. Today's Date:

Morning

(work towards continuing your night time dry fast up until at least 12pm)

Afternoon

(get hydrating with fresh fruit or even better slow juiced fruits/berries/melons)

Evening

(aim to wind down to a dry fast by around 6pm to 7pm)

Night

(work your way up to dry fasting from the evening until 12pm the following day)

Today's Notes (Highlights, Thoughts, Feelings, What Could You Improve On?)

"If you are struggling with hunger pangs in the early stages, try some dates or dried apricots, prunes, or raisins, with a cup of herbal tea.

8. Today's Date:

Morning
(work towards continuing your night time dry fast up until at least 12pm)

Afternoon
(get hydrating with fresh fruit or even better slow juiced fruits/berries/melons)

Evening
(aim to wind down to a dry fast by around 6pm to 7pm)

Night
(work your way up to dry fasting from the evening until 12pm the following day)

Today's Notes (Highlights, Thoughts, Feelings, What Could You Improve On?)

"Get into a routine of regularly buying fresh fruit (or grow your own if weather permits) to keep your supplies up."

---

9. Today's Date:

Morning

(work towards continuing your night time dry fast up until at least 12pm)

Afternoon

(get hydrating with fresh fruit or even better slow juiced fruits/berries/melons)

Evening

(aim to wind down to a dry fast by around 6pm to 7pm)

Night

(work your way up to dry fasting from the evening until 12pm the following day)

**Today's Notes (Highlights, Thoughts, Feelings, What Could
You Improve On?)**

*"Regularly remind yourself about the
great rewards and benefits that you will
experience from keeping up this detox."*

10. Today's Date:

Morning

(work towards continuing your night time dry fast up until at least 12pm)

Afternoon

(get hydrating with fresh fruit or even better slow juiced fruits/berries/melons)

Evening

(aim to wind down to a dry fast by around 6pm to 7pm)

Night

(work your way up to dry fasting from the evening until 12pm the following day)

Today's Notes (Highlights, Thoughts, Feelings, What Could You Improve On?)

"Keep your teeth brushed and flossed regularly – at least twice a day to keep them healthy for your fruit sessions. You will notice an improvement in your dental health with this raw/fruit diet."

11. Today's Date:

Morning
(work towards continuing your night time dry fast up until at least 12pm)

Afternoon
(get hydrating with fresh fruit or even better slow juiced fruits/berries/melons)

Evening
(aim to wind down to a dry fast by around 6pm to 7pm)

Night
(work your way up to dry fasting from the evening until 12pm the following day)

Today's Notes (Highlights, Thoughts, Feelings, What Could You Improve On?)

"Be motivated by the vision of becoming an example for others to learn from and follow."

12. Today's Date:

Morning
(work towards continuing your night time dry fast up until at least 12pm)

Afternoon
(get hydrating with fresh fruit or even better slow juiced fruits/berries/melons)

Evening
(aim to wind down to a dry fast by around 6pm to 7pm)

Night
(work your way up to dry fasting from the evening until 12pm the following day)

Today's Notes (Highlights, Thoughts, Feelings, What Could You Improve On?)

"Embrace your achievements and wonderful results – feel and appreciate the difference within you as a result of this new routine."

13. Today's Date:

Morning
(work towards continuing your night time dry fast up until at least 12pm)

Afternoon
(get hydrating with fresh fruit or even better slow juiced fruits/berries/melons)

Evening
(aim to wind down to a dry fast by around 6pm to 7pm)

Night
(work your way up to dry fasting from the evening until 12pm the following day)

"Buy fruit in bulk where possible so you have ample supplies for a week or two in advance. If in a hot climate, you could even freeze your fruit or make ice lollies out of it (crush & freeze)."

14. Today's Date:

Morning

(work towards continuing your night time dry fast up until at least 12pm)

Afternoon

(get hydrating with fresh fruit or even better slow juiced fruits/berries/melons)

Evening

(aim to wind down to a dry fast by around 6pm to 7pm)

Night

(work your way up to dry fasting from the evening until 12pm the following day)

Today's Notes (Highlights, Thoughts, Feelings, What Could You Improve On?)

"Stay as busy as you can during the daytime. Creating a busy routine makes it easier to manage your diet."

---

15. Today's Date:

Morning
(work towards continuing your night time dry fast up until at least 12pm)

Afternoon
(get hydrating with fresh fruit or even better slow juiced fruits/berries/melons)

Evening
(aim to wind down to a dry fast by around 6pm to 7pm)

Night
(work your way up to dry fasting from the evening until 12pm the following day)

Today's Notes (Highlights, Thoughts, Feelings, What Could You Improve On?)

"Complete your fruit and fasting routine with a group of friends/family/colleagues so you can all support one another."

16. Today's Date:

Morning

(work towards continuing your night time dry fast up until at least 12pm)

Afternoon

(get hydrating with fresh fruit or even better slow juiced fruits/berries/melons)

Evening

(aim to wind down to a dry fast by around 6pm to 7pm)

Night

(work your way up to dry fasting from the evening until 12pm the following day)

"Monitor your urine regularly. Urinate in a jar and leave overnight. If you see a thick cloud of white sediment (success!), your kidneys are filtering acids out."

17. Today's Date:

Morning
(work towards continuing your night time dry fast up until at least 12pm)

Afternoon
(get hydrating with fresh fruit or even better slow juiced fruits/berries/melons)

Evening
(aim to wind down to a dry fast by around 6pm to 7pm)

Night
(work your way up to dry fasting from the evening until 12pm the following day)

Today's Notes (Highlights, Thoughts, Feelings, What Could You Improve On?)

"Have genuine love and care for yourself. If craving junk food, affirm positive inner talk ("if I eat this, I won't feel good so leave it out")".

18. Today's Date:

Morning
(work towards continuing your night time dry fast up until at least 12pm)

Afternoon
(get hydrating with fresh fruit or even better slow juiced fruits/berries/melons)

Evening
(aim to wind down to a dry fast by around 6pm to 7pm)

Night
(work your way up to dry fasting from the evening until 12pm the following day)

Today's Notes (Highlights, Thoughts, Feelings, What Could You Improve On?)

"Filter out unwanted acids with this alkaline water-dense fruits protocol."

19. Today's Date:

Morning
(work towards continuing your night time dry fast up until at least 12pm)

Afternoon
(get hydrating with fresh fruit or even better slow juiced fruits/berries/melons)

Evening
(aim to wind down to a dry fast by around 6pm to 7pm)

Night
(work your way up to dry fasting from the evening until 12pm the following day)

Today's Notes (Highlights, Thoughts, Feelings, What Could You Improve On?)

"Look out for white cloud/sediment (acids) in your urine to confirm kidney filtration."

20. Today's Date:

Morning
(work towards continuing your night time dry fast up until at least 12pm)

Afternoon
(get hydrating with fresh fruit or even better slow juiced fruits/berries/melons)

Evening
(aim to wind down to a dry fast by around 6pm to 7pm)

Night
(work your way up to dry fasting from the evening until 12pm the following day)

Today's Notes (Highlights, Thoughts, Feelings, What Could You Improve On?)

.

"Infections emerge in an acidic environment"

21. Today's Date:

Morning
(work towards continuing your night time dry fast up until at least 12pm)

Afternoon
(get hydrating with fresh fruit or even better slow juiced fruits/berries/melons)

Evening
(aim to wind down to a dry fast by around 6pm to 7pm)

Night
(work your way up to dry fasting from the evening until 12pm the following day)

Today's Notes (Highlights, Thoughts, Feelings, What Could You Improve On?)

"Any deficiencies that you may have will disappear once you have cleansed your clogged up gut/colon, kidneys and various other eliminative organs."

22. Today's Date:

Morning

(work towards continuing your night time dry fast up until at least 12pm)

Afternoon

(get hydrating with fresh fruit or even better slow juiced fruits/berries/melons)

Evening

(aim to wind down to a dry fast by around 6pm to 7pm)

Night

(work your way up to dry fasting from the evening until 12pm the following day)

Today's Notes (Highlights, Thoughts, Feelings, What Could You Improve On?)

"Dependant on how deeply you detox yourself, you could even eliminate any genetic weaknesses that you may have inherited."

23. Today's Date:

Morning
(work towards continuing your night time dry fast up until at least 12pm)

Afternoon
(get hydrating with fresh fruit or even better slow juiced fruits/berries/melons)

Evening
(aim to wind down to a dry fast by around 6pm to 7pm)

Night
(work your way up to dry fasting from the evening until 12pm the following day)

Today's Notes (Highlights, Thoughts, Feelings, What Could You Improve On?)

"Keep focused on your detox. Even past injuries / trauma are all repairable for good."

24. Today's Date:

Morning
(work towards continuing your night time dry fast up until at least 12pm)

Afternoon
(get hydrating with fresh fruit or even better slow juiced fruits/berries/melons)

Evening
(aim to wind down to a dry fast by around 6pm to 7pm)

Night
(work your way up to dry fasting from the evening until 12pm the following day)

Today's Notes (Highlights, Thoughts, Feelings, What Could You Improve On?)

"If you suffer from ongoing sadness / depression, a deep detox will support your mental health. You will soon notice a positive change in your mood."

25. Today's Date:

Morning

(work towards continuing your night time dry fast up until at least 12pm)

Afternoon

(get hydrating with fresh fruit or even better slow juiced fruits/berries/melons)

Evening

(aim to wind down to a dry fast by around 6pm to 7pm)

Night

(work your way up to dry fasting from the evening until 12pm the following day)

Today's Notes (Highlights, Thoughts, Feelings, What Could You Improve On?)

"Have your fruits/juices throughout the day. As the evening approaches, start to dry fast – your body wants to rest and heal from this point on."

26. Today's Date:

Morning

(work towards continuing your night time dry fast up until at least 12pm)

Afternoon

(get hydrating with fresh fruit or even better slow juiced fruits/berries/melons)

Evening

(aim to wind down to a dry fast by around 6pm to 7pm)

Night

(work your way up to dry fasting from the evening until 12pm the following day)

Today's Notes (Highlights, Thoughts, Feelings, What Could You Improve On?)

"The kidneys dislike proteins but really appreciate juicy fruits like melons, berries, citrus fruits, pineapples, mangoes, apples, grapes."

27. Today's Date:

Morning
(work towards continuing your night time dry fast up until at least 12pm)

Afternoon
(get hydrating with fresh fruit or even better slow juiced fruits/berries/melons)

Evening
(aim to wind down to a dry fast by around 6pm to 7pm)

Night
(work your way up to dry fasting from the evening until 12pm the following day)

Today's Notes (Highlights, Thoughts, Feelings, What Could You Improve On?)

"Healing is very easy. There's no need to complicate it. Keep it simple and you will see results."

28. Today's Date:

Morning
(work towards continuing your night time dry fast up until at least 12pm)

Afternoon
(get hydrating with fresh fruit or even better slow juiced fruits/berries/melons)

Evening
(aim to wind down to a dry fast by around 6pm to 7pm)

Night
(work your way up to dry fasting from the evening until 12pm the following day)

Today's Notes (Highlights, Thoughts, Feelings, What Could You Improve On?)

"Keep your body in an alkaline state as this is where regeneration takes place."

29. Today's Date:

Morning
(work towards continuing your night time dry fast up until at least 12pm)

Afternoon
(get hydrating with fresh fruit or even better slow juiced fruits/berries/melons)

Evening
(aim to wind down to a dry fast by around 6pm to 7pm)

Night
(work your way up to dry fasting from the evening until 12pm the following day)

Today's Notes (Highlights, Thoughts, Feelings, What Could You Improve On?)

"A daily enema with boiled water (cooled down) will support your detox greatly."

30. Today's Date:

Morning
(work towards continuing your night time dry fast up until at least 12pm)

Afternoon
(get hydrating with fresh fruit or even better slow juiced fruits/berries/melons)

Evening
(aim to wind down to a dry fast by around 6pm to 7pm)

Night
(work your way up to dry fasting from the evening until 12pm the following day)

**Today's Notes (Highlights, Thoughts, Feelings, What Could
You Improve On?)**

*"Have your iris' read by an iridologist that
works with Dr Bernard Jensen's system."*